Helpful Lyme

Disease Cookbook

Top Recipes to Heal Your Body

BY: Valeria Ray

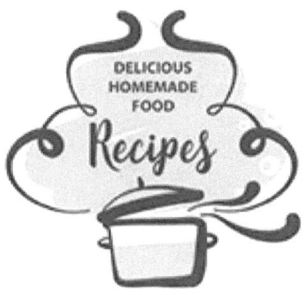

License Notes

A Special Reward for Purchasing My Book!

Thank you, cherished reader, for purchasing my book and taking the time to read it. As a special reward for your decision, I would like to offer a gift of free and discounted books directly to your inbox. All you need to do is fill in the box below with your email address and name to start getting amazing offers in the comfort of your own home. You will never miss an offer because a reminder will be sent to you. Never miss a deal and get great deals without having to leave the house! Subscribe now and start saving!

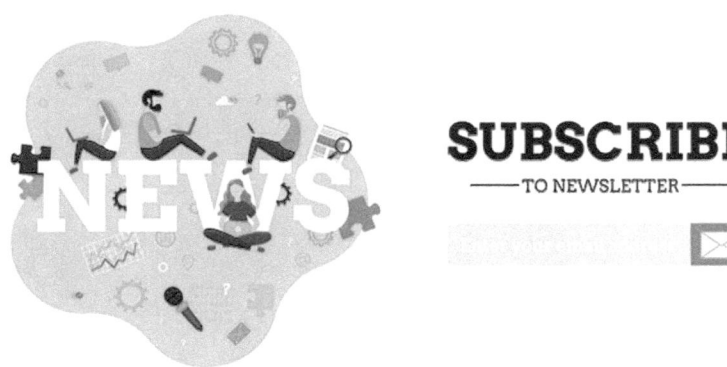

https://valeria-ray.gr8.com

Contents

Recipe 1: Loaded Cauliflower Casserole

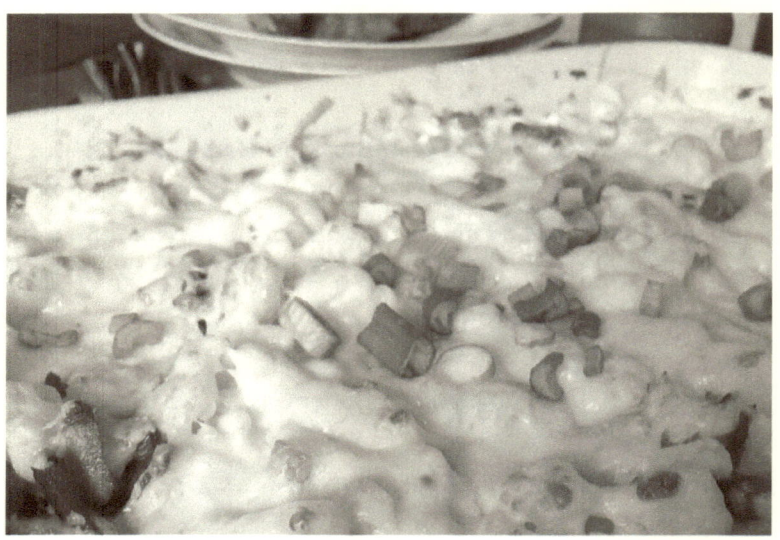

This is another healthy and filling casserole dish you can make whenever you are craving something on the healthier side.

Yield: 6 to 8 servings

Cooking Time: 35 minutes

List of Ingredients:

- 2 pounds of cauliflower florets
- 8 ounces of sharp cheddar cheese, shredded and evenly divided
- 8 ounces of Monterey jack cheese, shredded and evenly divided
- 8 ounces of cream cheese, soft
- 4 Tablespoons of heavy whipping cream
- 1 ½ cups of green onions, thinly sliced
- 6 bacon slices, cooked and crumbled
- 1 clove of garlic, grated
- Dash of salt and black pepper

MMMMMMMMMMMMMMMMMMMMMMMMMMMMMMMM

Methods:

1. Preheat the oven to 350 degrees.

2. In a steamer, steam the cauliflower florets for 5 minutes or until soft.

3. In a bowl, add in 6 ounces of shredded cheddar cheese, 6 ounces of the shredded Monterey jack cheese, soft cream cheese and heavy whipping cream. Sir well until creamy in consistency.

4. Add in the thinly sliced green onions, cooked bacon pieces and grated garlic. Stir well until evenly incorporated.

5. Set this mixture aside.

6. Add the steamed cauliflower into the cheese mix. Stir well until evenly mixed. Season with a dash of salt and black pepper.

7. Pour into a casserole dish. Sprinkle the remaining shredded cheddar and Monterey jack cheese over the top.

8. Cover with a sheet of aluminum foil.

9. Place into the oven to bake for 25 minutes. Remove the foil and continue to back for 2 to 3 minutes or until browned on the top.

10. Remove and serve immediately.

Recipe 2: Gluten Free Chicken Enchiladas

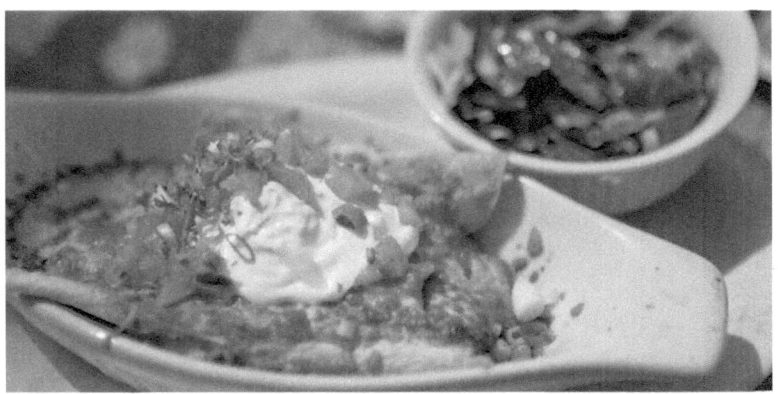

These delicious chicken enchiladas are incredibly flavorful and topped off with a gluten free sauce, it will leave you feeling full for several hours.

Yield: 8 servings

Cooking Time: 55 minutes

List of Ingredients:

- 8 ounces of cream cheese, soft
- 1, 8 ounce can of green chiles, chopped
- 1, 15 ounce can of white beans, drained
- 1 yellow onion, chopped
- ½ Tablespoons of extra virgin olive oil
- 2 chicken breasts, cooked and shredded
- 1, 14 ounce can of green enchilada sauce
- ¼ teaspoons of powdered garlic
- 2/3 cup of sour cream
- ¼ teaspoons of salt
- 8 to 10 gluten free tortillas
- 12 ounces of Monterey jack cheese, shredded

MMMMMMMMMMMMMMMMMMMMMMMMMMMMMMMMMM

Methods:

1. In a saucepan set over medium to high heat, add in the olive oil and chopped yellow onion. Cook for 5 minutes or until soft.

2. Add in the cream cheese into a stand mixer. Beat on the lowest setting until creamy in consistency. Add in the can of green chiles and can of white beans. Continue to mix until smashed lightly.

3. Add 2/3 of the onion mix into the cream cheese mix. Stir well to incorporate.

4. Place the saucepan with the remaining onion mix over medium to high heat. Add in the can of green enchilada sauce, powdered garlic, sour cream and dash of salt. Stir well to mix and allow to come to a boil. Cook for 2 to 3 minutes or until smooth in consistency. Remove and set aside.

5. Preheat the oven to 350 degrees.

6. Pour 1/3 of the enchilada sauce mix into a baking dish.

7. Heat the tortillas in a separate skillet for 30 seconds or until soft.

8. In each tortilla, add 1 to 2 tablespoons of the chicken mix. Sprinkle some of the shredded Monterey jack cheese over the filling. Roll the tortillas tightly and place into the baking dish with the seam sides facing down.

9. Pour the remaining sauce over the top of the enchiladas. Sprinkle the remaining Monterey jack cheese over the sauce.

10. Place into the oven to bake for 35 to 40 minutes.

11. Remove and cool for 5 minutes before serving.

Recipe 3: Healthy Turkey and Spinach Meatballs

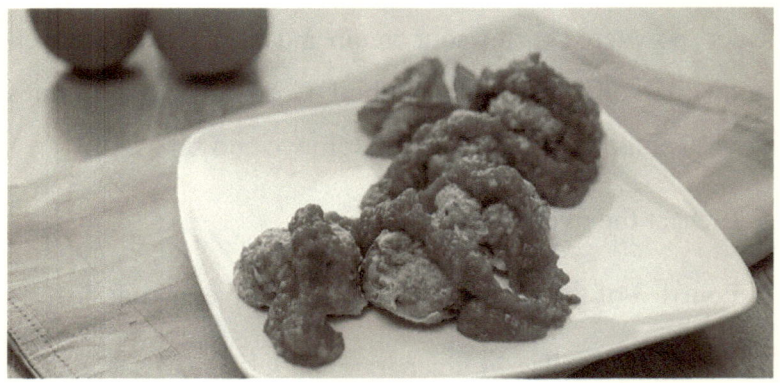

Make this Lyme Disease friendly meatballs during your next lunch or dinner party. These tasty appetizers are so tasty, I guarantee your friends and family will be begging you for the recipe.

Yield: 8 servings

Cooking Time: 35 minutes

List of Ingredients:

- 2 Tablespoons of extra virgin olive oil
- 1 onion, chopped
- 2 cloves of garlic, minced
- 1 teaspoon of salt
- ½ teaspoons of black pepper
- ¼ teaspoons of dried thyme
- ½ teaspoons of dried oregano
- ¼ to ½ teaspoons of crushed red pepper flakes, optional
- 1, 16-ounce pack of spinach, chopped
- 2 Tablespoons of Worcestershire sauce
- 1/3 cup of chicken broth
- 2 ½ pounds of lean ground turkey
- ¾ cup of breadcrumbs
- 2 eggs, beaten

MMMMMMMMMMMMMMMMMMMMMMMMMMMMMMMM

Methods:

1. Preheat the oven to 400 degrees. Grease a baking sheet with cooking spray.

2. In a frying pan set over medium to high heat, add in the olive oil. Add in the chopped onion, minced garlic, dried thyme, dried oregano and crushed red pepper flakes. Season with a dash of salt and black pepper. Cook for 5 minutes or until the onions are soft.

3. Add in the pack of spinach and toss well to mix.

4. Add in the Worcestershire sauce and chicken broth. Stir well to mix. Cook for 10 minutes or until the liquid is evaporated. Remove and set aside to cool completely.

5. In a bowl, add in the ground turkey, breadcrumbs and 1 of the beaten eggs. Stir well to mix. Pour the spinach mix into the bowl. Stir well with your hands until mixed.

6. Shape the meat mix into 1 inch balls. Place onto the baking sheet.

7. Place into the oven to bake for 20 minutes or until cooked through.

8. Remove and serve immediately.

Recipe 4: Gluten Free White Cake

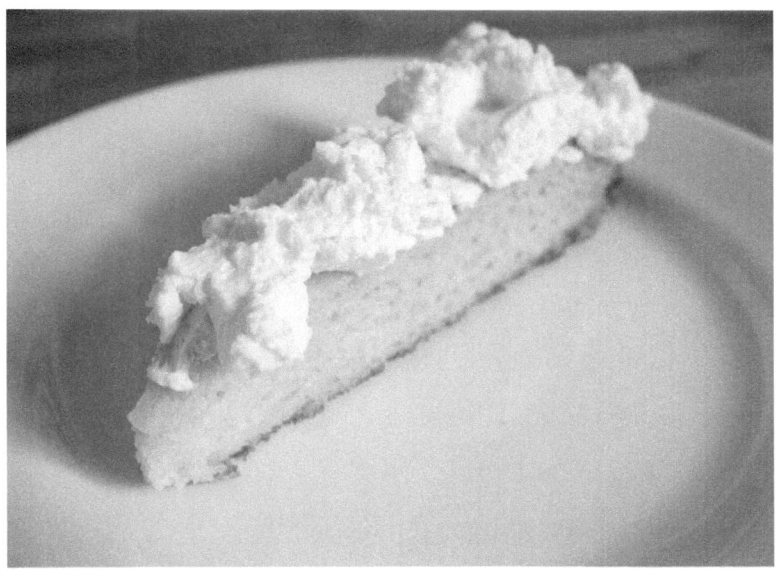

This is an incredibly soft and most white cake that is perfect to make regardless of the occasion. Serve with your favorite gluten-free icing.

Yield: 16 servings

Cooking Time: 1 hour

List of Ingredients:

- 1 ½ cups of brown rice flour
- 2/3 cup of potato starch
- 1/3 cup of tapioca starch
- ½ teaspoons of salt
- 1 tablespoon of baker's style baking powder
- 1 teaspoon of xanthan gum
- 4 eggs, beaten
- 1 cup of butter, melted and completely cooled
- 2 cups of white sugar
- 1 cup of buttermilk
- 1 teaspoon of pure vanilla
- 1 teaspoon of almond extract

MMMMMMMMMMMMMMMMMMMMMMMMMMMMMMM

Methods:

1. Preheat your oven to 350 degrees. Grease wo cake pan with butter. Line the bottom of each cake pan with a sheet of parchment paper.

2. In a bowl, add in the brown rice flour, potato starch, tapioca starch, salt, xanthan gum and baker's style baking powder. Stir well to mix.

3. In a separate bowl, add in the white sugar and beaten eggs. Beat with an electric mixer until creamy in consistency. Add into the flour mix. Stir well until mixed.

4. Add in the buttermilk, cooled butter, pure vanilla and almond extract. Beat again until just mixed.

5. Pour into the cake pans.

6. Place into the oven to bake for 35 to 40 minutes or until cooked through.

7. Remove and cool for 30 minutes before serving.

Recipe 5: Gluten Free Strawberries and Cream Cake

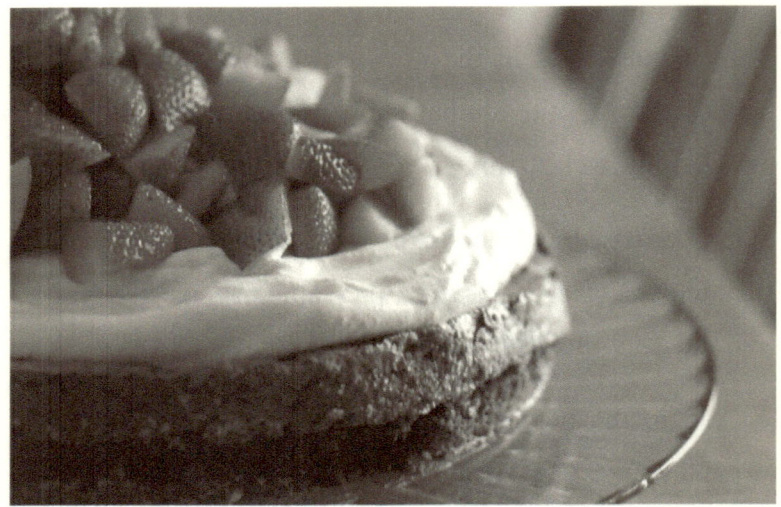

This is another tasty gluten free cake recipe you can prepare for those special occasions that you need to celebrate.

Yield: 10 servings

Cooking Time: 40 minutes

List of Ingredients:

- 2 cups of gluten free all-purpose flour
- 1 teaspoon of baker's style baking powder
- ½ teaspoons of baker's style baking soda
- ¼ teaspoons of salt
- ½ cup of butter, soft
- 1 ¾ cups of white sugar
- 4 egg whites
- 1 teaspoon of pure vanilla
- 2/3 cup of whole milk
- 2/3 cup of plain Greek yogurt

Ingredients for the filling:

- 2 cups of strawberries, thinly sliced
- 1 to 2 teaspoons of white sugar

Ingredients for the whipped cream:

- ¼ cup of powdered sugar
- 1 teaspoon of pure vanilla
- 1 pint of heavy whipping cream

MMMMMMMMMMMMMMMMMMMMMMMMMMMMMMMM

Methods:

1. Heat up the oven to 350 degrees. Grease three cake pans with baking spray. Place a round sheet of parchment paper into each pan.

2. In a bowl, add in the all-purpose flour, baker's style baking powder, baker's style baking soda and a dash of salt. Beat with an electric mixer or until creamy in consistency. Add in the

white sugar and continue to beat until smooth.

3. Add in the egg whites, pure vanilla, flour mix, whole milk and yogurt. Continue to beat on the lowest setting until evenly mixed.

4. Pour the batter among the cake pans.

5. Place into the oven to bake for 20 to 25 minutes or until baked through. Remove and set aside to cool completely.

6. In a bowl, add in the strawberries and white sugar for the filling. Stir well to mix and set aside for later use.

7. Prepare the whipped cream. In a separate bowl, add in the heavy whipping cream, powdered sugar and pure vanilla. Beat with a mixer until peaks begin to form on the surface.

8. Place one of the cakes onto a plate. Spread ½ cup of the whipped cream over the cake. Add a layer of half of the strawberries. Repeat with a second cake. Place the third cake on the top. Spread the remaining cream over the top.

9. Garnish with whole strawberries.

10. Serve immediately.

Recipe 6: Gluten Free Cinnamon Rolls

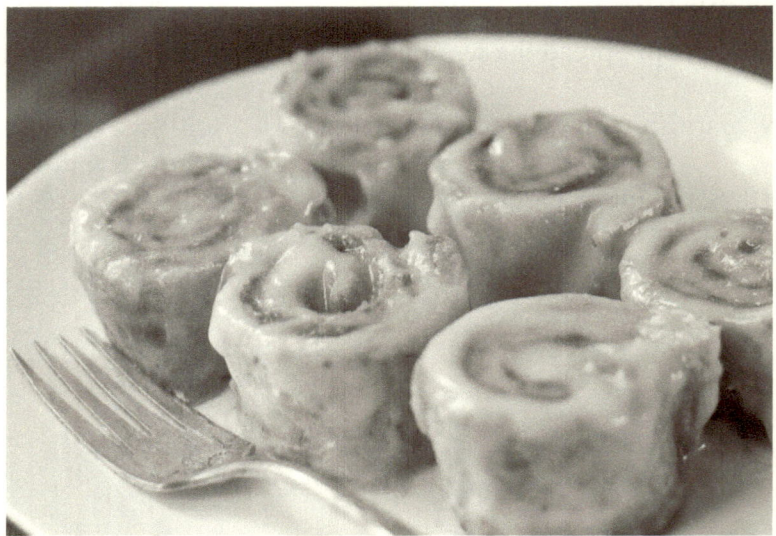

If you want to spoil your family with something special early in the morning, then this is the perfect dish for you to make.

Yield: 36 servings

Cooking Time: 2 hours

Ingredients for the dough:

- 1 quart of whole milk
- 1 cup of vegetable oil
- 1 cup of white sugar
- 4 ½ teaspoons of active dry yeast
- 8 ½ cups of gluten free flour
- 1 teaspoon of baker's style baking powder
- 1 teaspoon of baker's style baking soda
- 1 tablespoon of salt

Ingredients for the filling:

- 1 ½ cup of butter, melted
- ¼ cup of powdered cinnamon
- 2 cups of white sugar
- Ingredients for the icing:
- 8 ounces of cream cheese, soft
- 1 cup of whole milk
- 1 teaspoon of pure vanilla
- 2 pounds of powdered sugar

MMMMMMMMMMMMMMMMMMMMMMMMMMMMMMMMM

Methods:

1. Prepare the dough. In a saucepan set over medium heat, add in the whole milk, vegetable oil and white sugar. Stir well to mix. Cook for 3 minutes or until frothy. Remove and set aside to cool.

2. Sprinkle the dry yeast over the milk mix. Stir well to mix. Set aside to sit for 1 minute.

3. In a bowl, add the 8 cups of gluten free flour. Pour the milk mix into the bowl and stir well until mixed.

4. Cover the dough and set aside to rest for 1 hour.

5. To the dough, add the salt, remaining ½ cup of gluten free flour, baking powder and soda. Stir well until just mixed.

6. Divide the dough in half and place onto a flat surface. Roll into a rectangle that is 24 by 10 inches in size. Roll until ½ an inch in thickness.

7. Pour ¾ cup of melted butter onto the dough and spread evenly over the surface. Sprinkle 1 cup of white sugar and 1/8 cup of powdered cinnamon over the top.

8. Roll the dough into a tight log. Slice into 1 ½ inch slices. Place the slices into the greased baking dish.

9. Preheat the oven to 375 degrees. Cover and set the rolls aside to rest for 20 minutes.

10. Place into the oven to bake for 10 to 15 minutes or until golden brown. Remove and set aside to cool for 5 minutes.

11. Prepare the icing. In a bowl, add the cream cheese and whole milk. Beat with an electric mixer until smooth in consistency. Add in the pure vanilla and powdered sugar. Continue to beat until smooth in consistency.

12. Pour the icing over the rolls. Serve immediately.

Recipe 7: Broccoli and Quinoa Casserole

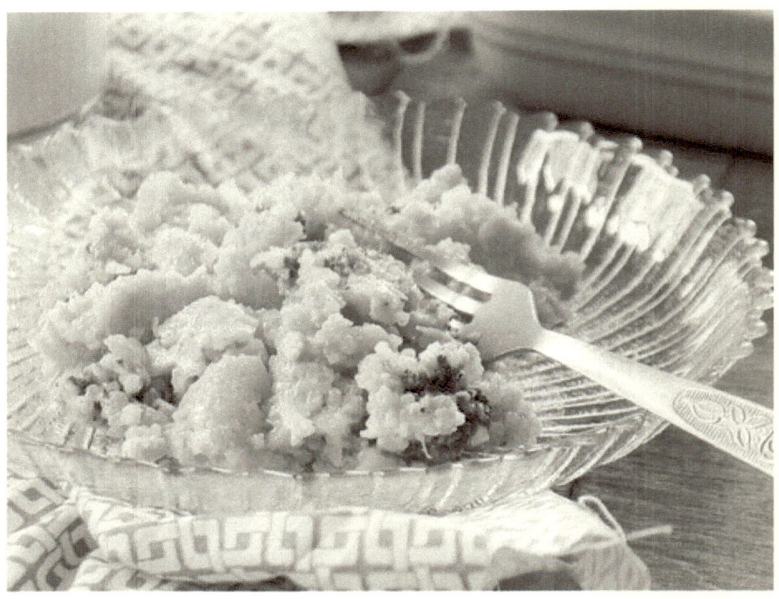

This is a healthy and comforting dish you can make whenever you have the need to spoil yourself.

Yield: 8 servings

Cooking Time: 30 minutes

List of Ingredients:

- 1 cup of quinoa
- 1 head of broccoli, cut into florets
- 2 Tablespoons extra virgin olive oil, evenly divided
- 1/3 cup of panko breadcrumbs
- 3 chicken breasts, boneless, skinless and thinly sliced
- Dash of salt and black pepper
- 2 Tablespoons of butter, soft
- 2 Tablespoons all-purpose flour
- 2 cups of 2% milk
- 1 ½ cups of cheddar cheese, shredded and evenly divided
- 1/3 cup of Greek yogurt

MMMMMMMMMMMMMMMMMMMMMMMMMMMMMMMMMMM

Methods:

1. Preheat the oven to 350 degrees. Grease a baking dish with cooking spray.

2. In a saucepan set over medium to high heat, add in 2 cups of the water. Add in the quinoa and cook according to the directions on the package. During the last 5 minutes or cooking, add in the broccoli. Cook for the remaining 5 minutes.

3. In a skillet set over medium to high heat, add in 1 tablespoon of olive oil. Add in the panko breadcrumbs. Cook for 3 minutes or until toasted. Remove and set aside.

4. In the same skillet, add in another tablespoon of the olive oil.

5. Season the chicken breasts with a dash of salt and black pepper. Add into the skillet. Cook for 4 minutes on both sides or until cooked through. Remove and rest for 10 minutes. Chop into small pieces.

6. In the same skillet, add in the soft butter. Add in the all-purpose flour and whisk until smooth in consistency. Cook for 1 minute. Add in the 2% milk and continue to cook for 5 minutes or until thick in consistency.

7. Add in the cooked quinoa, broccoli, cooked chicken pieces, 1 cup of the shredded cheddar cheese and Greek yogurt. Stir well until evenly mixed. Season with a dash of salt and black pepper.

8. Spread into the baking dish. Sprinkle the remaining ½ cup of shredded cheddar cheese over the top.

9. Place into the oven to bake for 5 minutes or until melted.

10. Remove and sprinkle the breadcrumbs over the top. Serve immediately.

Recipe 8: Lyme Disease Friendly Texas Dinner Rolls

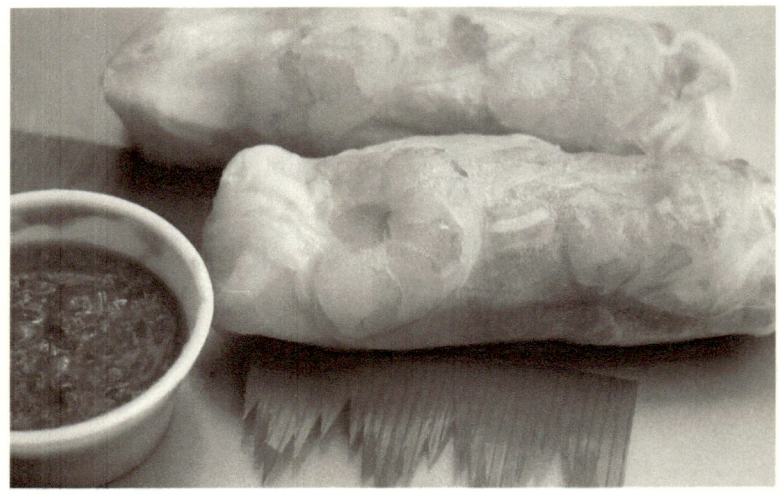

These Texas style dinner rolls are incredibly soft and fluffy, you will want to make these rolls nearly every night for dinner.

Yield: 12 servings

Cooking Time: 25 minutes

List of Ingredients:

- 3 cups of gluten free bread flour, extra for sprinkling
- 2 teaspoons of active yeast
- ¼ cup of white sugar
- 1 teaspoon of salt
- 1 cup + 1 tablespoon of pineapple juice
- 4 Tablespoons of butter soft
- 1 cup of warm whole milk
- 3 Tablespoons of butter, soft
- 1 tablespoon of honey

MMMMMMMMMMMMMMMMMMMMMMMMMMMMMMMMM

Methods:

1. In a bowl of a stand mixer, add in the glute free bread flour, active yeast and white sugar. Beat well until evenly mixed.

2. Add in the salt, 4 tablespoons of soft butter and pineapple juice. Beat on the lowest setting until a dough begins to form.

3. Place the dough onto a flat surface and knead for 5 minutes or until the dough is smooth in consistency.

4. Transfer into a greased bowl. Cover and set aside to rest for 12 hours.

5. Place the dough onto a large baking sheet and place the dough onto it. Roll the dough into a large 6 by 8 inch rectangle. Cut the dough rectangle into 12, 2 inch rolls.

6. Cover and set aside to rest for 45 minutes.

7. In a small bowl, add in the 3 tablespoons of soft butter and honey. Microwave for 30 seconds or until the butter melts. Whisk to mix. Brush this mixture over the top of the rolls.

8. Place into the oven to bake for 10 to 12 minutes or until gold.

9. Remove and cool for 5 minutes before serving.

Recipe 9: Vegan Cookie Dough Cheesecake Bites

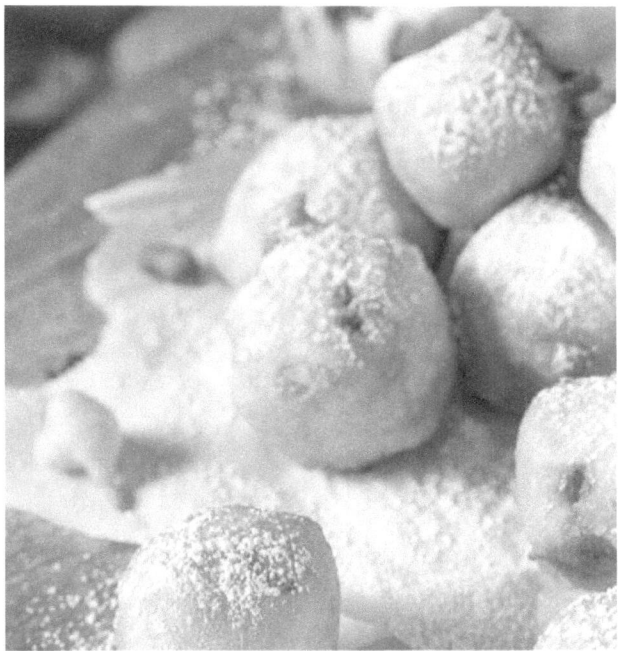

This is the perfect dish for you to make whenever you are craving something on the sweeter side. It is so delicious, even the pickiest of children won't be able to resist these bites once they get a taste of it.

Yield: 18 servings

Cooking Time: 24 hours

Ingredients for the crust:

- 1 cup of dates, pitted, soaked and drained
- ¼ cup of unsweetened coconut, shredded
- 1 cup of peanuts, dry roasted
- 1 cup of almonds
- 1 teaspoon of pure vanilla
- ¼ cup of ground flaxseed
- ¼ cup of water
- ¼ cup of dark chocolate chips

Ingredients for the topping:

- ¼ cup of coconut oil
- ¼ cup of agave nectar
- 1 teaspoon of pure vanilla
- 3 cups of cashews, soaked and drained
- ½ of a lemon, juice only
- ¼ cup of chocolate chips, for topping

MMMMMMMMMMMMMMMMMMMMMMMMMMMMMMMMMM

Methods:

1. In a food processor, add the ingredients for the topping except for the chocolate chips. Pulse on the highest setting until smooth in consistency. Transfer into a bowl and set aside.

2. In the same processor, add in the ingredients for the crust except for the chocolate chips. Pulse on the highest setting until smooth in consistency. Transfer into a separate bowl.

3. In the bowl with the crust mix, add in the dark chocolate chips. Fold gently until incorporated.

4. Grease a baking pan with cooking spray. Press the crust into the baking dish.

5. Spread the topping over the top. Sprinkle ¼ cup of the remaining chocolate chips over the topping.

6. Cover and place into the fridge to chill overnight.

7. Remove. Slice into bars and serve.

Recipe 10: Flourless Breakfast Cinnamon Bun Cake

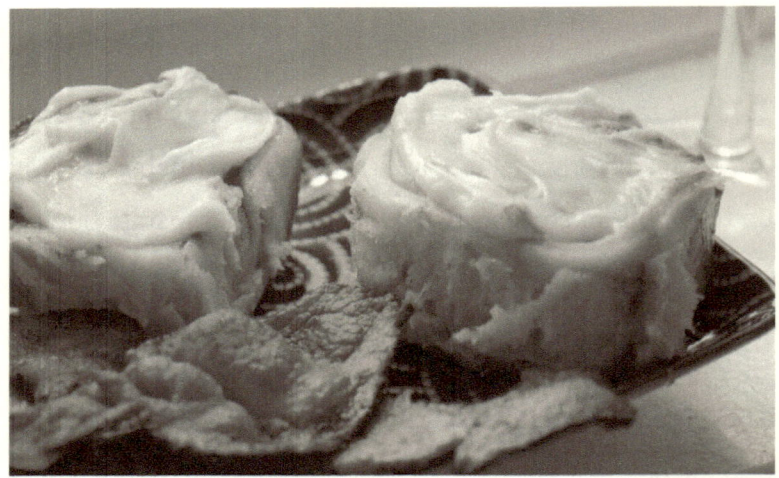

Just as the name implies, this is the perfect Lyme disease friendly cake dish you can serve early in the morning to give your body the much-needed energy you need.

Yield: 4 servings

Cooking Time: 35 minutes

Ingredients for the cake:

- 2 cups of gluten free rolled oats, ground
- ½ cup of coconut palm sugar
- 1 tablespoon of baker's style baking powder
- 1 tablespoon of Saigon cinnamon
- Dash of sea salt
- 1 cup of milk, dairy free
- 1 flax egg
- 1 teaspoon of pure vanilla
- 6 Tablespoons of almond butter, melted

Ingredients for the frosting:

- 1, 8-ounce box of cream cheese, dairy free
- 2 Tablespoons of sweetener
- 1 tablespoon of Saigon cinnamon

MMMMMMMMMMMMMMMMMMMMMMMMMMMMMMMMMM

Methods:

1. Preheat the oven to 350 degrees. Grease a loaf pan with a cooking spray.

2. Prepare the cake. In a bowl, add in the ground rolled oats, coconut palm sugar, baker's style baking powder, Saigon cinnamon and dash of sea salt. Stir well to mix.

3. In a separate bowl, add in the dairy free milk, pure vanilla and flax egg. Stir well to mix. Pour into the ground oat mix and stir well until evenly mixed.

4. Add in the melted almond butter. Stir well to evenly incorporate.

5. Pour into the greased loaf pan.

6. Place into the oven to bake for 25 to 30 minutes or until golden and baked through.

7. Remove and cool completely before serving.

Recipe 11: Salmon with Sriracha Sauce

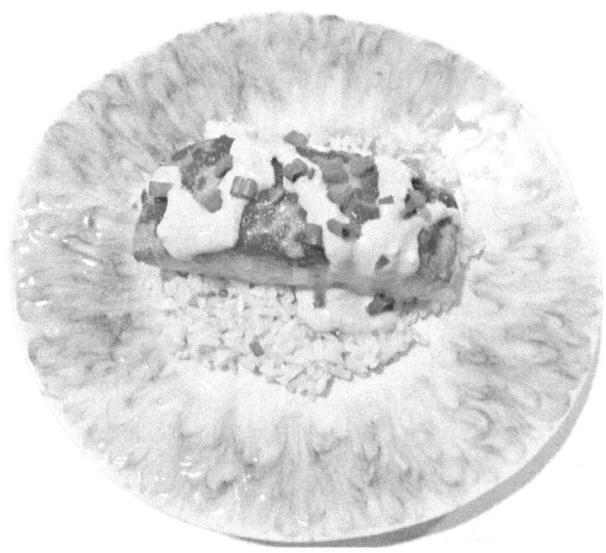

This is the perfect dish for you to make whenever you are craving something on the spicy side. Make this whenever you are craving homemade seafood.

Yield: 4 servings

Cooking Time: 15 minutes

List of Ingredients:

- ½ of a lime, juice and zest only
- 1 tablespoon of maple syrup
- 1 ½ teaspoons of Sriracha sauce
- ½ teaspoons of sea salt
- 1 ¼ pounds of salmon fillet, skin removed
- 2 Tablespoons of cilantro, chopped

MMMMMMMMMMMMMMMMMMMMMMMMMMMMMMMMMMM

Methods:

1. Preheat the oven to 425 degrees.

2. In a bowl, add in the fresh lime juice, fresh lime zest, maple syrup and Sriracha sauce. Season with a dash of salt. Whisk well to mix.

3. Place the salmon fillet into a baking dish. Pour the lime mix over the top.

4. Place the salmon into the oven to roast for 15 minutes or until cooked through.

5. Remove and serve immediately with the chopped cilantro.

Recipe 12: Gluten Free Lemon and Dijon Mustard Shrimp Pasta

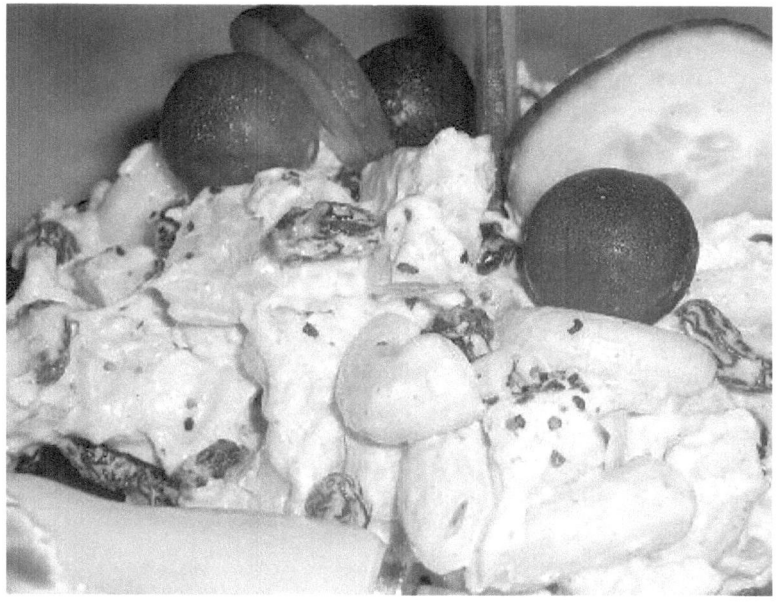

This is the perfect dish to make during your next Italian pasta night. It is so delicious, you will become hooked after your first bite.

Yield: 4 servings

Cooking Time: 40 minutes

List of Ingredients:

- ¼ cup of extra virgin olive oil
- 2 teaspoons of lemon zest, grated
- ¼ cup of lemon juice
- 2 Tablespoons of gluten free Dijon mustard
- 5 cloves of garlic, minced and evenly divided
- 8 ounces of Gluten free fettucine pasta
- 1 tablespoon of extra virgin olive oil, evenly divided
- 1 tablespoon of ghee, evenly divided
- 1 ½ pounds of shrimp, peeled and deveined
- 1 ½ teaspoons of sea salt
- 1 teaspoon of crushed red pepper flakes
- 1/3 cup of chives, snipped

MMMMMMMMMMMMMMMMMMMMMMMMMMMMMMMMM

Methods:

1. Prepare the sauce. In a bowl, add in ¼ cup of the extra virgin olive oil, fresh lemon zest, fresh lemon juice, Dijon mustard and 1 of the minced cloves of garlic. Stir well to mix.

2. Prepare the fettucine pasta according to the directions on the package.

3. In a skillet set over medium to high heat, add in 1 tablespoon of olive oil and 1 tablespoon of ghee. Add in the remaining cloves of garlic. Cook for 30 seconds.

4. Season the shrimp with a dash of salt and crushed red pepper flakes. Add into the skillet. Cook for 2 to 3 minutes or until brown. Transfer onto a plate and set aside.

5. Pour the sauce into the skillet. Cook for 1 minute.

6. Add the shrimp back into the skillet. Toss to mix. Add the chives and toss again.

7. Remove and serve immediately.

Recipe 13: Gluten Free Cheddar Bay Biscuits

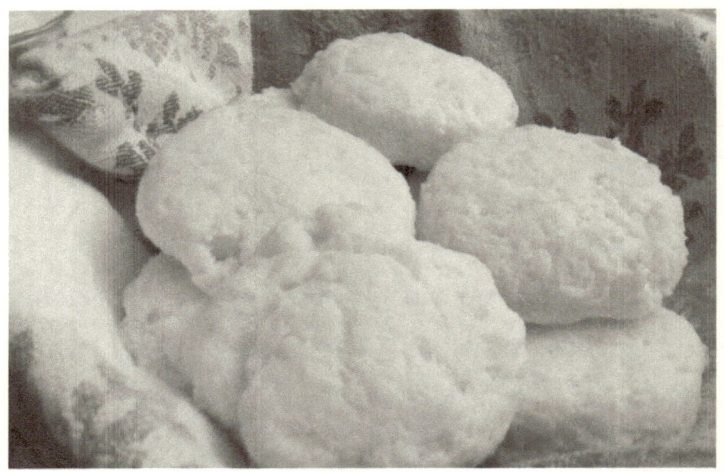

These light and flaky cheddar bay biscuits taste just like the gluten variety, just healthier. They are incredibly easy to put together, you can have them ready in just a matter of minutes.

Yield: 10 servings

Cooking Time: 30 minutes

List of Ingredients:

- 2 cups of all-purpose gluten free flour
- 1 teaspoon of xanthan gum
- ¼ cup of cornstarch
- 1 tablespoon of baker's style baking powder
- ½ teaspoons of salt
- 1 teaspoon of powdered garlic
- 6 ounces of sharp cheddar cheese, grated
- 2 Tablespoons of flat leaf parsley, chopped
- 8 Tablespoons of butter, cold and cut into small pieces
- 1 cup of buttermilk
- 2 Tablespoons of butter, melted

MMMMMMMMMMMMMMMMMMMMMMMMMMMMMMMMM

Methods:

1. Heat up the oven to 375 degrees. Place a sheet of parchment paper onto a baking sheet.

2. In a bowl, add the gluten free flour, xanthan gum, cornstarch, baker's style baking powder, dash of salt and powdered garlic. Whisk well until evenly mixed.

3. Add in the grated cheddar cheese, butter pieces and 1 tablespoon of parsley. Toss well to mix.

4. Add in the buttermilk and continue to mix until a dough begins to form.

5. Divide the dough into 10 pieces. Roll the pieces into smooth balls. Place onto the baking sheet and flatten slightly.

6. Transfer into the freezer to chill for 10 minutes or until firm.

7. In a bowl, add in the remaining ½ teaspoon of powdered garlic, remaining 1 tablespoon of chopped parsley and 2 tablespoons of melted butter. Stir well until evenly mixed. Brush onto the rolls.

8. Place into the oven to bake for 20 minutes or until browned.

9. Remove and set aside to cool for 5 minutes before serving.

Recipe 14: Gluten Free Chocolate Chip Cookies

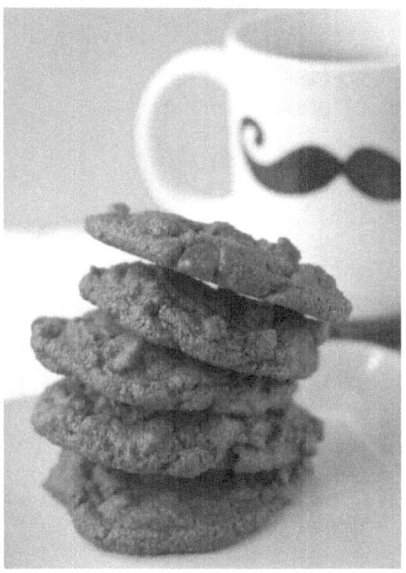

Make these delicious chocolate chip cookies whenever you are craving something packed with chocolate. Decadent and gluten free, these are perhaps the simplest cookies you will ever make.

Yield: 20 servings

Cooking Time: 4 hours and 30 minutes

List of Ingredients:

- 2 ¼ cups of all-purpose gluten free flour
- ½ teaspoons of xanthan gum
- 1 teaspoon of baker's style baking soda
- 1 teaspoon of salt
- 2 ounces of cream cheese, soft
- ¾ cups of butter, melted
- 1 cup of light brown sugar
- ½ cup of white sugar
- 1 ½ teaspoons of pure vanilla
- 2 egg yolks
- 2 cups of semi-sweet chocolate chips

MMMMMMMMMMMMMMMMMMMMMMMMMMMMMMMMMM

Methods:

1. In a bowl, add in the gluten free flour, xanthan gum, dash of salt and baker's style baking soda. Stir well to mix and set the mixture aside.

2. In the bowl of a stand mixer, add in the soft cream cheese, melted butter, light brown sugar and white sugar. Beat on the medium setting until creamy in consistency. Add in the pure vanilla and egg yolks. Beat again.

3. Add the flour mix and continue to mix until just mixed.

4. Add in the chocolate chips and fold gently until evenly incorporated.

5. Cover and set into the fridge to chill for 4 hours. Remove and set aside to rest for 15 minutes.

6. Preheat the oven to 375 degrees. Line two cookie sheets with sheets of parchment paper.

7. Using a cookie scoop, scoop the dough onto the cookie sheets, keeping them at least 1 inch a part.

8. Place into the oven to bake for 10 to 12 minutes.

9. Remove and cool for 10 minutes before serving.

Recipe 15: Gluten Free Floured Pumpkin Bread

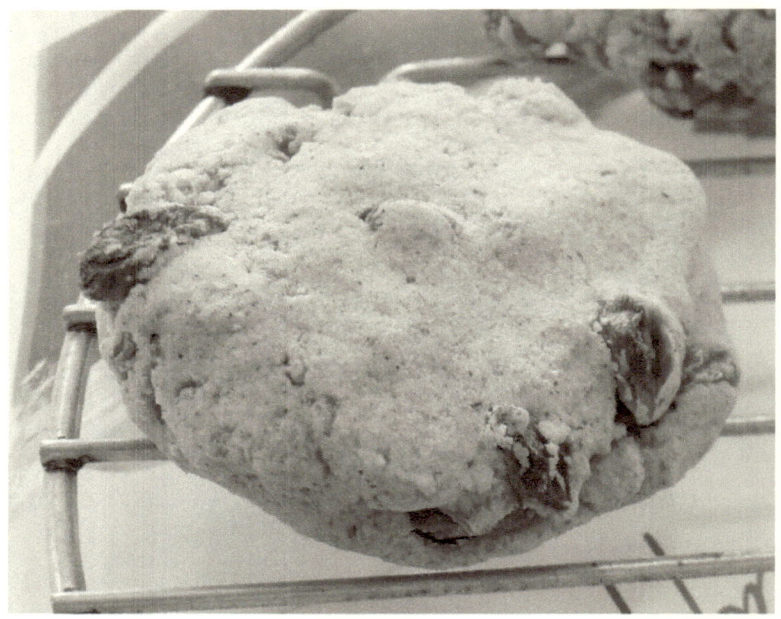

This is a delicious and gluten free bread you can make right in time for the holiday season. It is great to make even if you suffer from Lyme Disease.

Yield: 12 servings

Cooking Time: 1 hour and 5 minutes

Ingredients for the bread:

- ½ cup of maple syrup
- ½ cup of coconut oil, melted
- 4 eggs, beaten
- ¾ cup of pureed pumpkin
- 1 ½ teaspoons of pure vanilla
- ¾ cup of coconut flour
- ¾ teaspoons of baker's style baking soda
- ½ teaspoons of baker's style baking powder
- 1 ½ teaspoons of powdered cinnamon
- 1 teaspoon of pumpkin pie spice

Ingredients for the topping:

- 3 Tablespoons of coconut sugar
- 2 Tablespoons of coconut flour
- 2 Tablespoons of coconut oil, melted
- ½ teaspoons of powdered cinnamon
- 3 Tablespoons of walnuts, chopped

MMMMMMMMMMMMMMMMMMMMMMMMMMMMMMMM

Methods:

1. Heat up the oven to 350 degrees.

2. Prepare the bread. In a bowl, add the maple syrup, melted coconut oil and beaten eggs. Whisk well until evenly mixed. Add in the pureed pumpkin and pure vanilla. Whisk again until incorporated.

3. In a separate bowl, add the coconut flour, powdered cinnamon, pumpkin pie spice, baker's style baking powder and soda. Stir well until evenly mixed. Add in the pureed pumpkin mix and stir well until just mixed.

4. Line a loaf pan with a sheet of parchment paper. Pour the batter into the loaf pan.

5. Prepare the topping. In a bowl, add in the coconut sugar, coconut flour, melted coconut oil, powdered cinnamon and chopped walnuts. Stir well until just mixed and crumbly in consistency.

6. Sprinkle the crumb mix over the top of the batter.

7. Place into the oven to bake for 50 to 55 minutes or until baked through.

8. Remove and cool for 30 minutes before serving.

Recipe 16: Gluten Free Pull-Apart Dinner Rolls

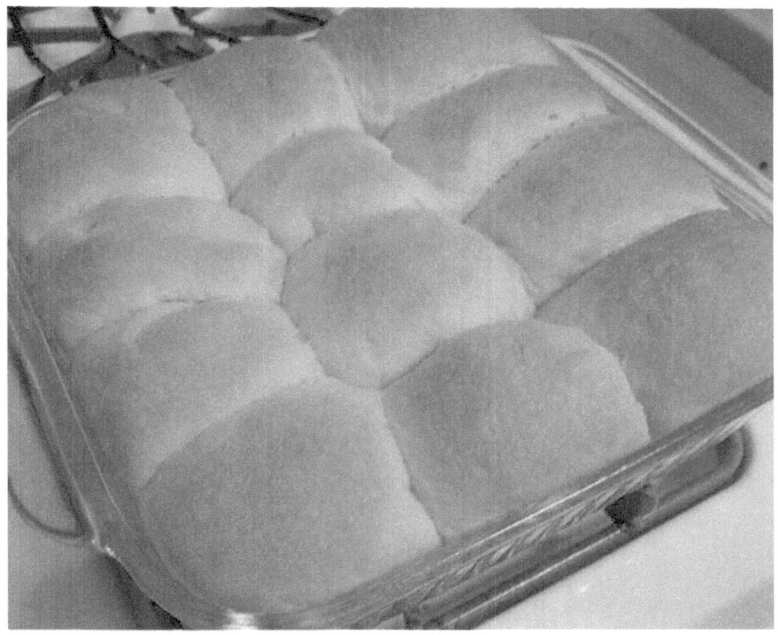

This is another dinner roll recipe that I know you will want to make as often as possible once you get a taste of them for yourself.

Yield: 6 servings

Cooking Time: 1 hour and 35 minutes

List of Ingredients:

- 2 ¾ cups of gluten free almond flour
- 1 ½ teaspoons of xanthan gum
- 2 teaspoons of active yeast
- ¼ cup of white sugar
- Dash of salt
- 1 cup of warm water
- 2 Tablespoons of butter, melted
- 1 egg, beaten
- 1 teaspoon of cider vinegar

MMMMMMMMMMMMMMMMMMMMMMMMMMMMMMMM

Methods:

1. In the bowl of a stand mixer, add the gluten free almond flour, xanthan gum, yeast, white sugar and dash of salt. Stir well to mix.

2. While the stand mixer is running, add in the water, melted butter, beaten egg and cider vinegar. Continue to mix until evenly mixed.

3. Grease a cake pan with cooking spray.

4. Add in scoops of the dough into the cake pan to form mounds.

5. Cover and set aside to rest for 45 minutes to 1 hour.

6. Preheat the oven to 400 degrees.

7. Place into the oven to bake for 25 to 30 minutes or until baked through.

8. Remove and brush the rolls with the melted butter. Serve immediately.

Recipe 17: Flourless Peanut Butter Cookies

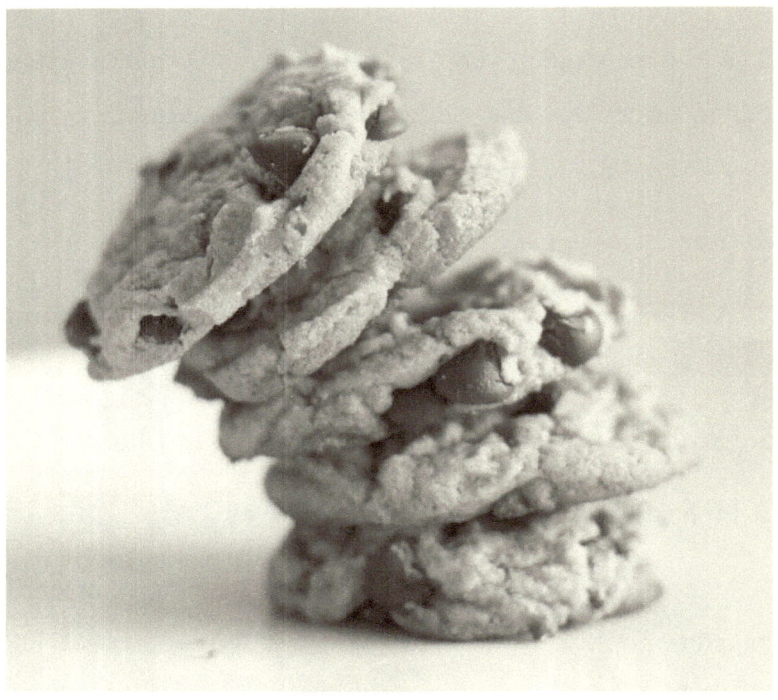

If you love the taste of peanut butter cookies, then this is one cookie dish that I know you will loves, especially if you are suffering from Lyme Disease.

Yield: 24 servings

Cooking Time: 25 minutes

List of Ingredients:

- 1 egg, beaten
- 1 cup of sweetener
- 1 teaspoon of baker's style baking powder
- ½ teaspoons of pure vanilla
- 1 cup of creamy peanut butter
- 1 teaspoon of water
- 1/3 cup of peanuts, chopped and optional

MMMMMMMMMMMMMMMMMMMMMMMMMMMMMMMM

Methods:

1. Heat up the oven to 350 degrees.

2. In a bowl, add in the beaten egg, sweetener, baker's style baking powder and pure vanilla. Use an electric mixer until evenly mixed.

3. In a separate bowl, add in the creamy peanut butter and water. Beat with the electric mixer until smooth in consistency?

4. Add in the chopped peanuts if you are using them. Stir well until evenly incorporated.

5. Spoon spoonfuls of the cookie dough onto a cookie sheet. Press down slightly.

6. Place into the oven to bake for 15 minutes or until browned.

7. Remove and cool for 5 minutes before serving.

Recipe 18: Coconut and Pecan Breakfast Bars

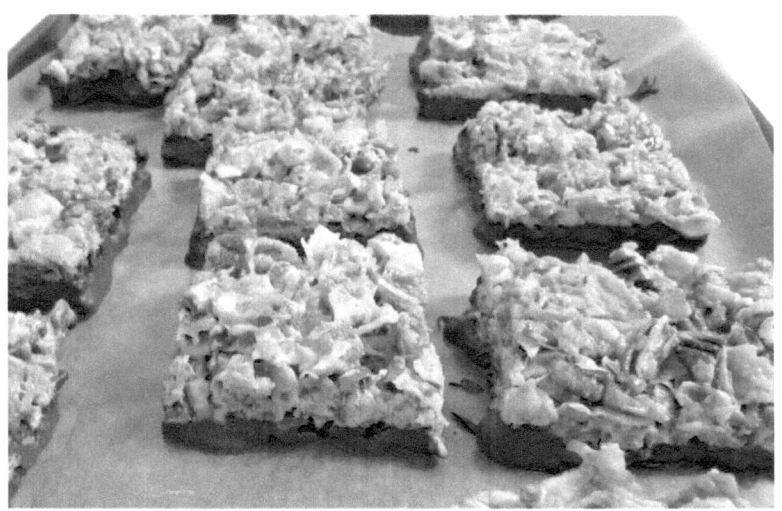

If you are looking for a healthy and delicious way to kick off your early morning, then these are the perfect breakfast bars for you to make.

Yield: 16 servings

Cooking Time: 30 minutes

List of Ingredients:

- Coconut oil, for greasing
- 2 eggs, beaten
- 1 banana, mashed
- ¼ cup of honey
- ½ teaspoons of pure vanilla
- 1/3 cup of coconut flour
- 1 cup of unsweetened coconut, shredded
- 4 Tablespoons of coconut milk
- ½ cup of pecans, chopped

MMMMMMMMMMMMMMMMMMMMMMMMMMMMMMM

Methods:

1. Preheat the oven to 350 degrees. Grease a baking dish with coconut oil.

2. In a bowl, add in the beaten eggs. Add in the mashed banana, honey and pure vanilla. Stir well to mix.

3. Add in the coconut flour, shredded unsweetened coconut and coconut milk. Stir well until just mixed.

4. Pour into the baking dish. Sprinkle the chopped pecans over the top.

5. Place into the oven to bake for 20 to 25 minutes or until baked through.

6. Remove and cool for 5 minutes. Slice into bars and serve immediately.

Recipe 19: Crustless Quiche

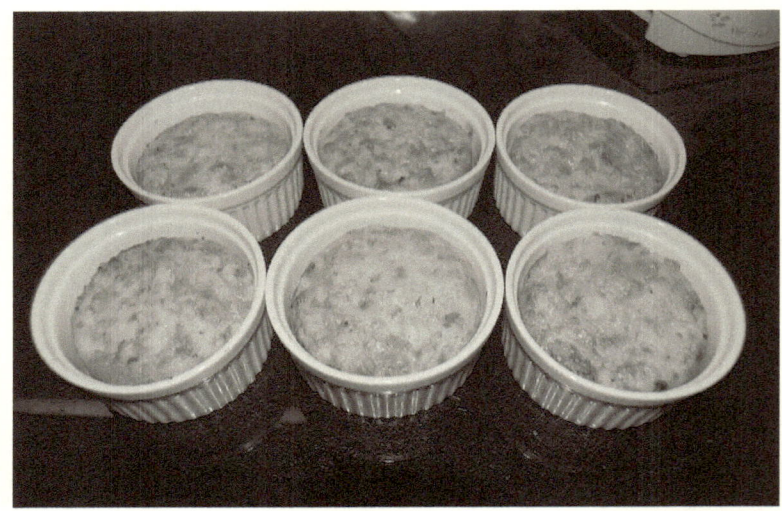

This is the perfect dish to make if you need to get away from the harmful gluten of most pie crusts. It is pretty simple to prepare and you will want to make it every night for dinner.

Yield: 6 servings

Cooking Time: 50 minutes

List of Ingredients:

- 1 pound of ground beef
- 1 onion, chopped
- 1 cup of mayonnaise
- 1 cup of whole milk
- 4 eggs, beaten
- 2 Tablespoons of cornstarch
- Dash of salt and black pepper
- 3 cups of cheddar cheese, shredded

MMMMMMMMMMMMMMMMMMMMMMMMMMMMMMMM

Methods:

1. In a skillet set over medium to high heat, add in the ground beef. Cook for 8 to 10 minutes or until browned.

2. Add in the chopped onion. Cook for 5 minutes or until soft.

3. In a bowl, add in the mayonnaise, whole milk, beaten eggs and cornstarch. Whisk well until evenly mixed.

4. Add the cooked beef and onions into the bowl with the eggs. Stir well to mix.

5. Pour into two greased pie pans.

6. Place into the oven to bake for 35 minutes at 350 degrees or until set.

7. Remove and serve immediately.

Recipe 20: Pumpkin Coffee Cake

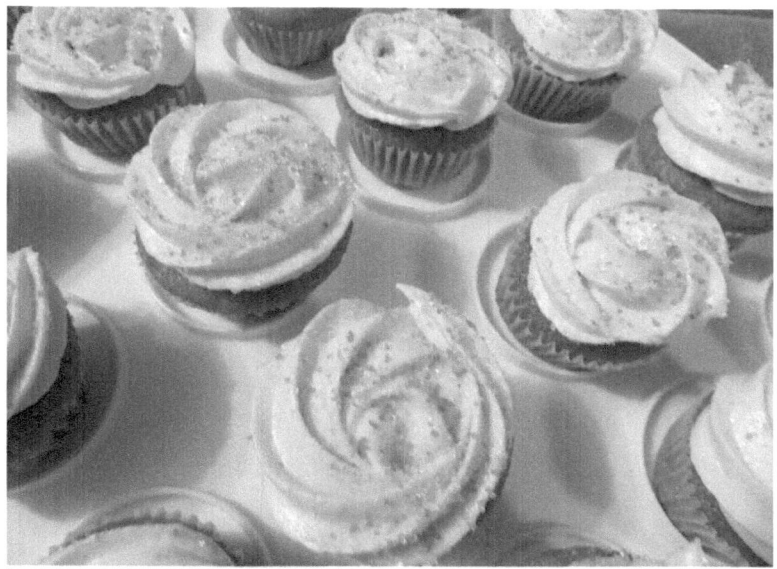

This is the perfect coffee cake to make right in time for the fall season. It is not only healthy for you, but it is incredibly delicious.

Yield: 9 servings

Cooking Time: 1 hour

Ingredients for the cake:

- ¼ cup coconut oil
- ¼ cup of maple syrup
- 1 cup of canned pumpkin
- 4 eggs, beaten
- ¼ cup of coconut sugar
- 1 cup of almond flour
- ¼ cup of coconut flour
- ½ teaspoons of baker's style baking soda
- 1 ½ teaspoons of pumpkin pie spice
- ½ teaspoons of powdered cinnamon
- ½ teaspoons of salt

Ingredients for the topping:

- ¼ cup of coconut flour
- ½ cup of ground almond flour
- 2 Tablespoons of coconut sugar
- ½ teaspoons of powdered cinnamon
- 2 Tablespoons of maple syrup
- 2 Tablespoons of coconut oil

MMMMMMMMMMMMMMMMMMMMMMMMMMMMMMM

Methods:

1. Preheat the oven to 325 degrees. Line a baking dish with a sheet of parchment paper.

2. Prepare the topping. In a bowl, add the ingredients for the topping. Stir well until crumbly in consistency. Set this mixture aside.

3. Prepare the cake. In a bowl, add in the ingredients for the cake. Stir until just mixed.

4. Pour into the greased baking dish. Top off with the crumb topping.

5. Place into the oven to bake for 45 to 50 minutes.

6. Remove and cool for 5 minutes before serving.

Recipe 21: Gluten Free French Butter Cake

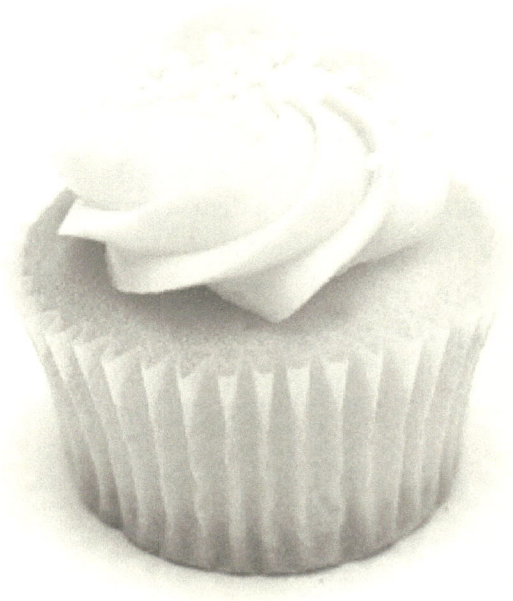

This Lyme Disease friendly dish is so delicious, I know you will want to make it every day, not just for those special occasions.

Yield: 8 servings

Cooking Time: 45 minutes

Ingredients for the bottom layer:

- 1 box of Pillsbury Gluten Free yellow cake mix
- ½ cup of butter, melted
- 2 eggs, beaten

Ingredients for the top layer:

- 1, 8-ounce block of cream cheese, soft
- 2 eggs, beaten
- 4 cups of powdered sugar
- 1 teaspoon of pure vanilla

MMMMMMMMMMMMMMMMMMMMMMMMMMMMMMMMM

Methods:

1. Heat up the oven to 350 degrees. Grease a baking dish with cooking spray.

2. Prepare the bottom layer. In the bowl, add the box of gluten free yellow cake mix, melted butter and 2 beaten eggs. Stir well to mix.

3. In a separate bowl, add in the ingredients for the top layer. Stir well until smooth in consistency.

4. Pour the cake mix into the baking dish. Spread the cream cheese mix over the top.

5. Place into the oven to bake for 35 to 40 minutes or until baked through.

6. Remove and set aside to cool completely before serving.

Recipe 22: Gluten Free Apple Muffins

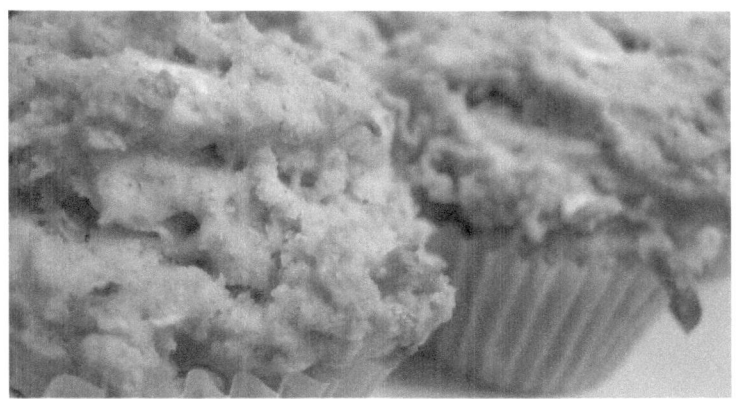

These incredibly moist apple muffins are made having an amazing texture and are one of the easiest muffins you can make.

Yield: 14 servings

Cooking Time: 35 minutes

Ingredients for the muffins:

- 2 cups of almond flour
- ¼ cup of coconut flour
- ½ teaspoons of salt
- 2 teaspoons of baker's style baking powder
- ½ teaspoons of baker's style baking soda
- 4 teaspoons of powdered cinnamon
- ½ teaspoons of ground ginger
- ½ teaspoons of ground nutmeg
- 3 eggs, beaten
- 2/3 cup of honey
- 1 ½ teaspoons of pure vanilla
- ½ cup of plain Greek yogurt
- 1 ½ cups of apples, peeled and chopped

Ingredients for the streusel:

- ¼ cup of almond flour
- 1 teaspoon of coconut flour
- ¾ teaspoons of powdered cinnamon
- 1 tablespoon of coconut oil
- 1 tablespoon of maple syrup
- Dash of salt
- 1/3 cup of pecans, chopped

Methods:

1. Preheat the oven to 425 degrees. Line a muffin pan with paper muffin liners.

2. Prepare the streusel. In a bowl, add in all of the ingredients for the streusel. Stir well until crumbly in consistency.

3. In a separate bowl, add in the ingredients for the muffins. Stir well until just mixed.

4. Fill the muffin cups ¾ of the way full with the muffin batter. Sprinkle the streusel over the top.

5. Place into the oven to bake for 5 minutes. Reduce the temperature of the oven to 350 degrees. Continue to bake for 10 to 15 minutes or until baked through.

6. Remove and set aside to cool for 10 minutes before serving.

Recipe 23: Gluten Free Breadsticks

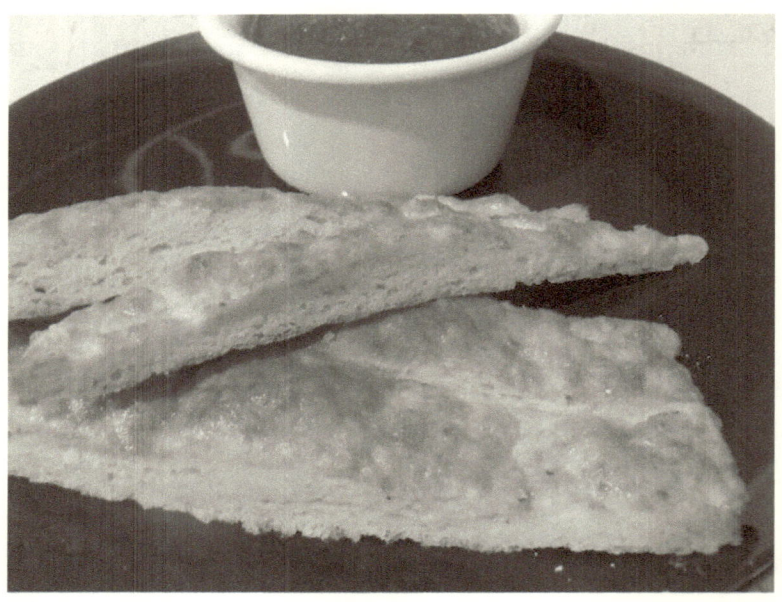

If you love the breadsticks from Olive Garden, then I know you won't be able to get enough of these breadsticks for yourself.

Yield: 12 servings

Cooking Time: 1 hour and 40 minutes

Ingredients for the dough:

- 4 ½ cups of gluten free bread flour, extra for sprinkling
- 2 teaspoons of instant yeast
- 2 Tablespoons of white sugar
- 2 teaspoons of salt
- 6 Tablespoons of butter, soft
- 1 ¼ cups + 2 Tablespoons of warm water

Ingredients for the garlic butter:

- 3 Tablespoons of butter, melted
- 1 teaspoon of garlic salt

MMMMMMMMMMMMMMMMMMMMMMMMMMMMMMM

Methods:

1. Prepare the dough. In a bowl of a stand mixer, add in the gluten free bread flour, instant yeast and white sugar. Stir well until evenly mixed. Add in the salt, butter and water. Continue to mix until evenly mixed.

2. Set the stand mixer to the knead setting. Knead for 5 minutes or until the dough is smooth in consistency.

3. Line a baking sheet with a sheet of parchment paper.

4. Divide the dough into 12 pieces. Shape each into rounds and shape into a rectangle that is ½ an inch in thickness and that is 4 inches long. Repeat and place onto the baking sheet.

5. Cover and set aside to rest for 1 hour and 25 minutes.

6. Preheat the oven to 375 degrees.

7. Place the breadsticks into the oven. Reduce the temperature of the oven immediately to 350 degrees. Bake for 5 minutes.

8. In a bowl, add the melted butter and garlic salt. Stir well until mixed. Brush onto the breadsticks. Place the breadsticks back into the oven to bake for 5 minutes or until golden.

9. Remove and brush again with the butter.

10. Remove and serve immediately.

Recipe 24: Lyme Diseases Friendly Chicken Tenders

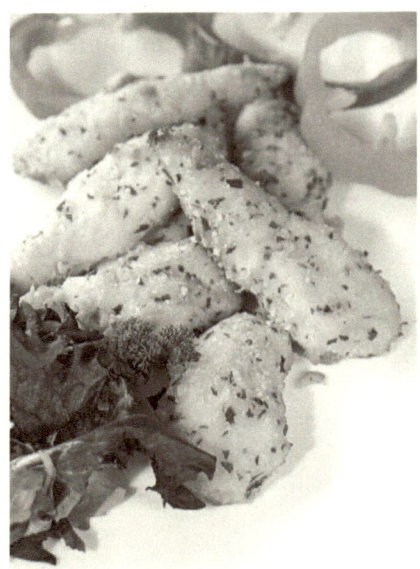

These delicious chicken tenders are so easy to make, I know you will want to make them over and over again. It is gluten free, so you don't have to worry about consuming it in the process.

Yield: 6 servings

Cooking Time: 20 minutes

List of Ingredients:

- 1 ½ pounds of chicken, organic and cut into thin strips
- 1/3 cup of coconut flour
- 2 eggs, beaten
- 1 tablespoon of cashew milk
- 1 cup of almond flour
- ½ teaspoons of salt
- ¼ teaspoons of black pepper
- ½ teaspoons of powdered garlic
- ½ teaspoons of powdered onion
- ¼ teaspoons of cayenne pepper, optional

MMMMMMMMMMMMMMMMMMMMMMMMMMMMMMMM

Methods:

1. Preheat the oven to 425 degrees. Line a baking sheet with a sheet of parchment paper.

2. In 3 shallow bowls, add the coconut flour into one and the almond flour, powdered garlic, powdered onion, cayenne pepper, dash of salt and dash of black pepper into the second bowl. Stir well to mix. In the third bowl, add the beaten eggs and the cashew milk. Whisk to mix.

3. Take the chicken strips and dip first into the coconut flour mix. Roll until coated on all sides. Dip into the egg mix. Then dredge in the almond flour mix until coated on all sides. Place onto the baking sheet.

4. Place into the oven to bake for 10 minutes. Flip and continue to bake for another 5 minutes.

5. Remove and cool for 5 minutes before serving.

Recipe 25: Breakfast Carrot Cake

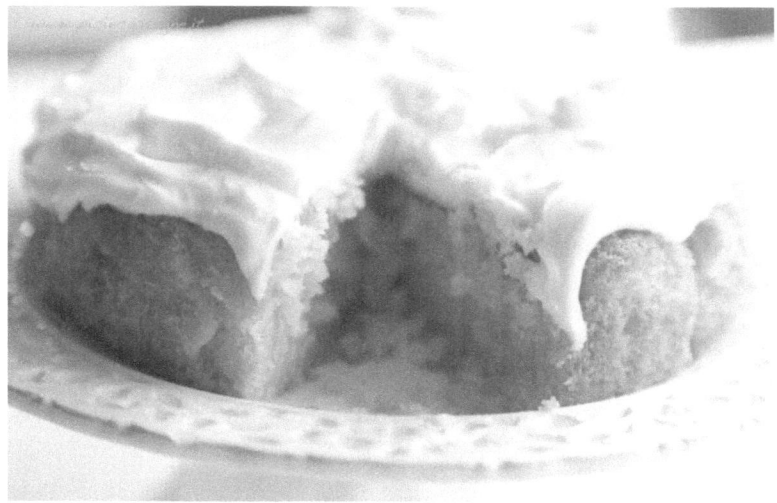

This is another delicious breakfast dish that you can make that is packed with plenty of protein, it will help to give you the energy you need to get you going in the morning.

Yield: 6 servings

Cooking Time: 40 minutes

List of Ingredients:

- 2 cups of gluten free oat flour
- ½ cup of sweetener
- 1 tablespoon of baker's style baking powder
- Dash of sea salt
- 1 carrot, grated
- 1 cup of milk, dairy free
- 1 flax egg
- 1 teaspoon of pure vanilla
- 6 Tablespoons of almond butter, melted

Ingredients for the frosting:

- 4 to 6 Tablespoons of coconut butter, melted
- 2 Tablespoons of sweetener
- Milk, dairy free and as needed for thinning

MMMMMMMMMMMMMMMMMMMMMMMMMMMMMMMMM

Methods:

1. Heat up the oven to 350 degrees. Grease a baking dish with cooking spray.

2. Prepare the carrot cake. In a bowl, add the dairy free milk, pure vanilla and flax egg. Stir well to mix.

3. Add in the gluten free oat flour, sweetener, baker's style baking powder, sea salt, grated carrot and melted almond butter. Stir well until just mixed.

4. Pour into the greased baking dish.

5. Place into the oven to bake for 25 to 30 minutes or until baked through.

6. Remove and set aside to cool for 5 minutes.

7. Prepare the frosting. In a separate small bowl, add in the melted coconut butter and sweetener. Add in as much dairy free milk you need to thin out the frosting to your desired consistency.

8. Spread the frosting over the top of the cake. Serve immediately.

About the Author

A native of Indianapolis, Indiana, Valeria Ray found her passion for cooking while she was studying English Literature at Oakland City University. She decided to try a cooking course with her friends and the experience changed her forever. She enrolled at the Art Institute of Indiana which offered extensive courses in the culinary Arts. Once Ray dipped her toe in the cooking world, she never looked back.

When Valeria graduated, she worked in French restaurants in the Indianapolis area until she became the head chef at one of the 5-star establishments in the area. Valeria's attention to taste and visual detail caught the eye of a local business person who expressed an interest in publishing her recipes. Valeria began her secondary career authoring cookbooks and e-books which she tackled with as much talent and gusto as her first career. Her passion for food leaps off the page of her books which have colourful anecdotes and stunning pictures of dishes she has prepared herself.

Valeria Ray lives in Indianapolis with her husband of 15 years, Tom, her daughter, Isobel and their loveable Golden Retriever, Goldy. Valeria enjoys cooking special dishes in her large, comfortable kitchen where the family gets involved in preparing meals. This successful, dynamic chef is an inspiration to culinary students and novice cooks everywhere.

••••••••• ● ● ● ● ● ●•••••••

Author's Afterthoughts

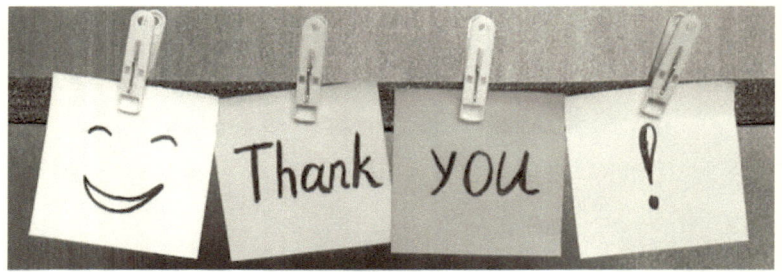

Thank you for Purchasing my book and taking the time to read it from front to back. I am always grateful when a reader chooses my work and I hope you enjoyed it!

With the vast selection available online, I am touched that you chose to be purchasing my work and take valuable time out of your life to read it. My hope is that you feel you made the right decision.

I very much would like to know what you thought of the book. Please take the time to write an honest and informative review on Amazon.com. Your experience and opinions will be of great benefit to me and those readers looking to make an informed choice.

With much thanks,

Valeria Ray

www.ingramcontent.com/pod-product-compliance
Lightning Source LLC
Chambersburg PA
CBHW020338290526
45785CB00005B/2083